MW00463742

CRYSTAL PROTECTION
from **5G** and
EMF POLLUTION

Barbara Newerla

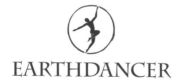

EARTHDANCER

AN INNER TRADITIONS IMPRINT

Second revised edition 2020, reprinted 2021
First edition 2010
Crystal Protection from 5G and EMF Pollution
Barbara Newerla

This English edition © 2020 Earthdancer GmbH
English translation © 2010 Astrid Mick
English translation of updated material © 2020 JMS books LLP
Editing by JMS books LLP (www.jmseditorial.com)

First English edition published in 2010 under the title
Protect Yourself from Electromagnetic Pollution

Originally published in German as
Heilsteine bei Elektrosmog – Was wirklich hilft und nützt
World © 2009 Neue Erde GmbH, Saarbrücken, Germany

Cover Design: Aaron Davis
Cover photography: 123RF.com
Typesetting and Layout: DesignIsIdentity.com
Typeset in News Gothic

Printed and bound in China by Reliance Printing Co., Ltd.

ISBN 978-1-64411-143-7 (print)
ISBN 978-1-64411-144-4 (ebook)

Published by Earthdancer, an imprint of Inner Traditions
www.earthdancerbooks.com, www.innertraditions.com

FSC
www.fsc.org
MIX
Paper from
responsible sources
FSC® C102842

Contents

Radiation has become a hot button topic as never before. The explosive rise in the private use of radio technology over the last few years is a matter of considerable concern. It raises the question of what effects it might have on people and their health, not to mention the digitalization that has taken place in every aspect of our lives, with similarly unpredictable results on individuals and society in general.

However, by the 1980s and the triumphant advent of the personal computer (first in our offices and then in our private spaces), many people were already concerned about the impact of radiation from computer monitor screens.

When Michael Gienger, Anja Gienger, and I started our crystal business in the early 1990s and the concept of crystal healing began to spread ever farther afield, it prompted us to think about using crystals to protect against radiation from screens. It soon became apparent that certain crystals seem particularly suitable for this purpose, and these are still considered the "classic" electromagnetic pollution crystals today. However, more has since been discovered about how, why, and in what ways they work. And over time we have learned that there are many more crystals that can help the human body to cope with the burden of exposure to this kind of radiation.

Unfortunately, there are equally a number of misunderstandings in circulation about the use of crystals to protect against electromagnetic pollution. I therefore very much hope that this book will bring clarity to, and shed light on, not only the possibilities, but also the limitations of using crystals for this purpose.

What Is Electromagnetic Pollution?

The term "electromagnetic pollution" refers to the radiation generated by all man-made electrical, magnetic, and electromagnetic "fields" that surround us in our homes, work places, and public spaces. We describe something as "polluting" when we believe it has detrimental effects on ourselves and/or our environment.

A "field" is the zone or space in which an electrical or magnetic force is active. In the case of a conventional iron magnet, for example, the field is the space in which the magnet can attract an object made of iron. In the case of an electrical or electromagnetic field, it is the zone in which the radiation emitted can exert a measurable effect on an object or a body. The strength of the field decreases as the distance between the source and the object increases, just as the damaging effects of electro-magnetic pollution decrease the farther away your body is from the source of the radiation.

These fields are generated whenever an electrical appliance is in use or a transmitter is transmitting.

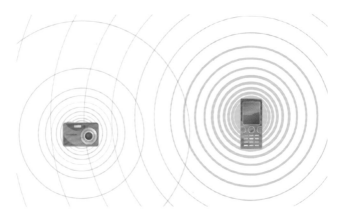

How and Where Is Electromagnetic Pollution Created?

Electromagnetic pollution is generated wherever an electrical current is flowing. Hence, it is present in the zones around the following sources:

✦ electrical devices or appliances

✦ cables or the leads of electrical appliances

✦ electric cables in walls and in sockets

✦ railway and tram lines

Electromagnetic pollution actually consists of two different types of field: magnetic and electrical.

The **magnetic field** is only generated when a current is flowing, in other words, when an appliance is switched on or is in standby mode.

The **electrical field** may unfortunately also be generated when an appliance is switched off, but its plug is still inserted in a socket.

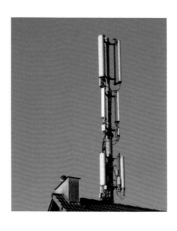

Electromagnetic pollution also occurs wherever radio waves are being emitted, for example, in the area around a transmitter. In this case, both electrical and magnetic fields are present, and the two become indistinguishable, creating what is known as an **electromagnetic field**. Depending upon its type and strength, the field's reach can vary from several hundred feet to many miles. Electromagnetic fields are generated around devices such as the following:

✦ radio and television transmitters

✦ cell phone transmission masts

✦ radar transmitters (near military installations and airfields)

✦ cordless telephones

✦ wifi routers, both at home and near public hotspots, laptops, and tablets with activated wifi

✦ dLAN networks (home plugs)

✦ wireless connections (Bluetooth) with a range of electrical devices, such as printers, keyboards, computers, and computer mice

✦ activated smartphones

✦ digital meters (electricity, gas, and water)

✦ smart devices that can be controlled from a smartphone or are linked to a smart home network

5G: The Next Generation of Radio Telephony

Any conversation about cell phone radiation these days is bound to include 5G. This is the abbreviation used for the fifth generation standard for cellular telephony; it will have far wider reaching effects on our lives, health, and life on this planet in general than we can currently even imagine.

The Industrial Revolution changed life for people in fundamental ways at the end of the 19th century, and now, in the first decades of the 21st century, 5G is laying the technological foundations for a transformation that could be termed the "Digital Revolution."

In so doing, 5G represents not just a clear and present threat to our freedom (it is paving the way for digital dictatorship and the end of any notion of privacy), but also a massive attack on our health.

If you think I am exaggerating, please read on. Further information may also be found on the internet and in relevant literature and documents. Although over the last 20 years or so, few people have taken much interest in the effects of exposure to cell phone radiation, it is no coincidence that groups protesting at the arrival of 5G are now springing up in many areas.

What Is 5G?

Toward the end of the 20th century, radio-based technologies began to develop at breakneck speed, ushering in the digitalization of every aspect of our lives; this ongoing evolution is now culminating in the introduction of the fifth generation (5G) of cellular telephony.

Data transmission was originally limited to voice and text-based communications (GSM, second generation, and so on), but with the advent of UMTS (Universal Mobile Telecommunications Service) and wifi standards (third generation), considerably more data could, for the

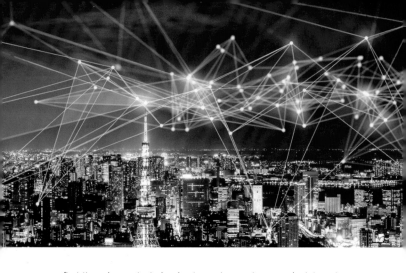

first time, be sent wirelessly at ever increasing speeds: internet access, images, and entire movies were almost universally available "on the go" via smartphones. The fourth generation (Long Term Evolution/LTE) was intended to provide even more capacity and speed, but is now already being overtaken by the fifth generation before the rollout of 4G has even been completed.

The Difference between 5G and Previous Cellular Telephony

✦ 5G uses additional, higher frequencies

However, transmitter range drops off significantly at higher frequencies and it is more difficult to penetrate physical obstacles such as buildings, walls, and trees. Achieving 100 percent network coverage will require **far more transmitters** and **far higher transmission output** in order to reach indoor areas. If 5G is to be universally available at some point in the future, a transmitter mast would have to be positioned every 165–330 feet.

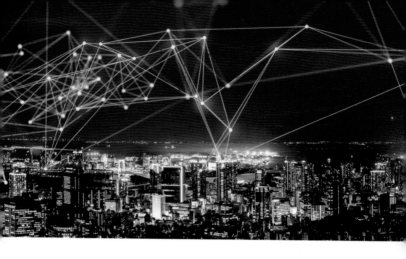

✦ Massive MIMO (Multiple Input, Multiple Output)

The number of antennae per transmitter site will also increase significantly, although the antennae themselves will be smaller. Until now, transmitters have contained 8 antennae. The antennae for 5G are considerably smaller, and each mast will contain 2 x 64 antennae, making a total of 128 per site, thus facilitating "beamforming."

✦ Beam forming

A technique in which a beam of radio waves can be targeted toward the end user device (a smartphone, for example), which is requesting or transmitting data at that particular time. The beam tracks users even when they move. This means that it is not broadcast across the whole area covered by the transmitter, but is instead directed specifically to where the relevant power is required.

✦ Satellites

There are plans to place some 20,000 satellites in orbit around Earth to provide broadband internet anywhere in the world via 5G.

The Potential Benefits of 5G

✦ Very high speeds.

✦ The possibility of supplying a great number of end user devices simultaneously.

✦ The IoT (Internet of Things): virtually all technological devices will be able to communicate (exchange data) with virtually all others. Smartphones, televisions, refrigerators, machinery, cars, PCs, and so on, will be able to "talk" to one another directly and exert an influence on each other.

✦ One network: the 5G standard will unite all previous cellular networks and their functions (including the various cell phone providers, TV and radio, wifi networks, and so on) in a single, large network. Unlimited, for better or for worse.

✦ Industry 4.0 (smart factories): 5G will enable further expansion of exclusively machine-controlled manufacturing. The automation and digital coordination of production processes will be increased.

✦ AI (artificial intelligence): the widespread use of intelligent machines will be made possible through the speed and ready availability—in no time at all—of large amounts of data. The need for human intervention is likely to become increasingly superfluous.

The Dangers of 5G: Health Consequences

As 5G is yet to become widespread and is still not available at anything like its full potential, we can at the moment only speculate about the specific repercussions of its broadcasting technology. However, one thing is fairly certain: radiation levels will rise exponentially in both private and public spaces.

Neither wifi nor second to fourth generation cell phone providers, from GSM (Global System for Mobile Communications) to LTE, are likely to disappear over the short term as 5G will not be able to replace all the other standards. This will lead to 5G antennae being added to all the existing transmitter sites.

To exploit 5G's full potential for the complete integration of every aspect of our lives into a network, at least one transmitter will be required every 330 feet. As a result, radio radiation will be more ubiquitous than ever before.

There is as yet no clarity at all about how indoor spaces are to be supplied with connectivity, however. The higher frequencies used by 5G are far less able to penetrate solid objects (such as walls, buildings...) than current cell phone signals. In order to deliver 5G to the interiors of buildings from outside, transmission levels will have to be increased to a substantial degree.

Furthermore, beamforming focuses transmission on the area where the radio waves are being used. It is precisely this that makes 5G so problematic as far as the exact measurement of radiation intensity is concerned. No one can say how much radiation will be generated at a particular point at any given time, and we don't yet have the capacity to measure 5G radiation at a specific location in a meaningful way. Because of beamforming, the intensity of the radiation can vary wildly and will depend on however many users there are requesting however much data at a particular location at a particular time.

The number of end user devices with an integrated transmitter will also increase (Internet of Things, smart home). General levels of radiation intensity will also continue to rise.

The use of higher frequencies will lead to certain plants and animals (especially insects), not to mention bacteria, suffering greater exposure. Human skin and eyes may also be particularly affected, as a function of the dimensions of the relevant physical structures, which themselves resonate with the corresponding wavelengths of the radiation.

In summary:

✦ Additional transmitters and an increased number of masts at more frequent intervals, combined with an increased number of antennae and more end user devices emitting radiation = greater exposure.

✦ Higher intensity due to the penetration of solid objects being poorer = greater exposure.

✦ Beamforming: it is impossible to calculate when or where radiation will be present, or how much there will be.

✦ Complete penetration into all aspects of life (areas that are free of radiation will more or less cease to exist).

✦ It will be almost impossible for an individual to control the radiation exposure within their home, not to mention work environment.

✦ Generally higher environmental damage as far as plants, animals, and certain parts of the human body are concerned, because of the higher frequencies and shorter wavelengths.

The Dangers of 5G: Individual and Social Consequences

Big data

The idea behind big data is to use as much data as possible to create a representation of a given current situation that is as precise as possible, and then to use this model to predict the future as accurately as possible. The main players in big data are now intelligent machines (artificial intelligence) rather than people, with the beneficiaries including governments, the economy, the international finance markets, and the military and secret services, to name but a few. Machines have been making decisions about buying and selling on trading floors for years, based on their ability to predict trends in the markets, and they now do this faster and better than any human ever could.

Intelligent machines control industrial manufacturing, analyze buyer behavior for large corporations, and monitor particular groups of people to identify what governments consider undesirable behavior before it can manifest itself in the real world.

The accuracy of the analysis of events—whether economic, military, or social—is based not only on the quality but also on the quantity of the data that can be applied. The amount of data available concerning individual people, and all the situations in our lives about which data can be exchanged in real time, will continue to grow exponentially with 5G, and with it the potential to predict the future behavior of individuals and to influence them appropriately.

The final obstacles to the unrestricted use and total integration of our personal data and the digital footprints that we leave in the internet fall away entirely with 5G. The speed and uniformity of the 5G network makes the prospect of total data fusion and data analysis by intelligent machines a possibility.

The personality profiles that are thus created reveal more about us than our friends and families could ever imagine, not to mention what

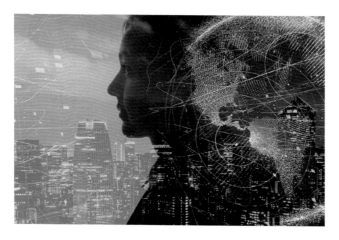

we imagine we know about ourselves. They build up a profile of who we are, our temperament and behavioral patterns, and can predict what we are likely to do or not do in certain situations, what scares us, along with what we desire and where our strengths and weaknesses lie.

Many find it hard to believe that a machine is capable of such things, but both the 2016 presidential election in America and the Brexit referendum in the UK, also in 2016, showed what is possible in this context; in both cases, suitable technology was used to:

✦ Locate people who had yet to make a final decision and were still "sitting on the fence."

✦ Influence these people—through their fears, inclinations, desires, and preferences—into making a particular voting choice by feeding them specific pieces of information.

The Consequences of Big Data in the Future

Knowledge is power, which means that data is power. Gathering data about us is in part given an attractive spin by disguising it as convenience; we are told that this information is a by-product of all the applications intended to make our lives simpler and more comfortable, relieving us of some of our "work" and making our lives safer.

Cameras are already ubiquitous, especially in larger cities, and more sensors will be introduced with 5G; detecting or measuring temperature, humidity, light, movement, pressure, and so on, these are the sensory organs of intelligent machines and the networked world.

No aspect of our lives will remain free of monitoring by sensors transmitting such data to another location for further processing. In many cases, we will have no control over who has access to specific data, nor indeed over who can gain access to it whenever they wish, not to mention the data we voluntarily publish to social media platforms and digital assistants, or via cell phone apps.

American whistleblower Edward Snowden has pointed the finger at what is already being done (and has been done over the last few years), and this potential to collect and analyze data will only increase with 5G. Don't imagine that at some point or other "they" will hold back. If it is technically possible, "they" will do it, and this kind of surveillance will no longer be the preserve of "just" the military, secret services, or state agencies, but will be undertaken by companies with commercial interests, organizations whose one true god is shareholder value.

In its ideal incarnation, your smart home will notice that you are on your way back from work and adjust the temperature accordingly to make it warm and cozy for your arrival. The oven will have switched itself on earlier to heat up the evening meal you have prepared. Your digital assistant will be playing your favorite tunes as you eat, while if you are not entirely sure what you would like to listen to, it will use physical data from your smart wristband to calculate your mood, comparing your general demeanor with similar situations in the past and making appropriate suggestions. Which is all well and good.

But what if the data that you constantly reveal through your buying habits on the internet, voluntarily surrender on social media platforms, or quantify through your smart home applications—your digital electricity, heating, and water meters, your wearable technology, or the apps on your smartphone—are collected, linked, and analyzed? It may ultimately produce a picture of you that is not to the liking of your government, health insurance provider, bank, or employer.

Your blood pressure is too high, you don't get enough sleep, and you don't take sufficient exercise, according to the electronic data-gatherer on your wrist that has become mandatory if you want to take out health insurance; it reminds you that if you do not change your lifestyle, your health insurance premium will unfortunately go up by 50 percent next month. What you do not know at this point is that your employer also has access to every last piece of data available about your lifestyle and, in the next round of downsizing, is going to place you on the list of people to whom it will soon be offering a redundancy agreement.

A little far-fetched? In the Western world it might be, for the moment at least, but China has already introduced a "social score" system; if you have too few points, your child will not be allowed to attend your chosen school, you won't get a new apartment, and your friends will shun you, since associating with someone lagging behind on the points system is detrimental to their own points tally. What will cause points to be deducted? Misdemeanors such as crossing the road on a red light, posting the wrong image at the wrong time, making critical remarks, paying bills late, turning up late for work more than once, taking too much sick leave. This is no joke. It is already grim reality.

It could not happen here? Really? Are you quite sure?

The driving force behind 5G, even in the USA and Europe, is politics. Yes, you read that right. It's not big business but the political world that is pressing for the rapid introduction of 5G, although as a technological standard, it is in some respects still in its infancy. The prospect of comprehensive surveillance is just too tempting, however.

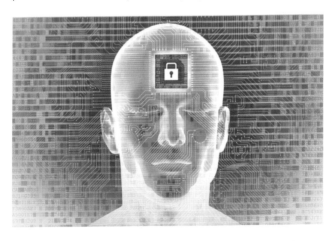

Other possible consequences of the digitalization of our world using 5G may include:

✦ Large-scale job losses and widening gulfs in society.

✦ The increasing involvement of every individual in virtual realities.

✦ Alienation from the natural world and natural resources.

✦ Complete dependence on digital devices and applications.

✦ Atrophy of cognitive capabilities (digital dementia).

5G, big data, and intelligent machines may be leading us into a future that is so bright, so perfect, and so secure that no hint of humanity, personal freedom, or individuality will remain.

What Can Be Done?

Be aware that all "smart" gadgets do the following:

✦ Constantly emit high-frequency, pulsed radio waves that can cause harm to you both mentally and physically (see page 22).

✦ Collect data, which it may pass on. This also includes practical apps on your smartphone. The data that they collect about you is the way you pay for these "free" little helpers.

Think carefully about what you reveal about yourself on the internet and on social networks.

As far as the physical and mental consequences of exposure to radiation are concerned, the same is true for 5G as it is for all other types of electrosmog: less is more. In other words, the less electrosmog there is, the better it is for your health.

You can find out more about this, and about what you can do to help yourself using healing crystals, in the following pages.

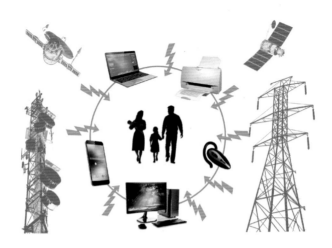

Does Electromagnetic Pollution Really Make You Sick?

It has been asserted repeatedly that electromagnetic pollution, and the pulsed electromagnetic radiation of cell phone traffic in particular, has no detrimental effects on the human body. This argument is based on the idea that the intensity of the radiation is far too low to create any warming or overheating of the tissues. What is really meant, however, is that there is no apparent damage; in other words, no visible damage, such as a burn to the skin.

There is no long-term research proving that being exposed to stress from electromagnetic pollution over a period of many years is safe. By contrast, researchers frequently find indications that the body can suffer major harm over the long term, even with low levels of intensity, and the World Health Organization has already classified this radiation as potentially carcinogenic. In addition, many people are discovering in their everyday lives that they are suffering from problems or issues that are undoubtedly connected with this kind of radiation; examples include problems that develop after a new cell phone mast has been erected or after having bought a digital cordless phone.

Our own practical experiences as building biologists deliver a clear message, as do the experiences of many of the people, including therapists and open-minded doctors, who work in the field of natural healing: electromagnetic pollution (as well as other stress factors in modern life) puts great strain on the human body; it facilitates and possibly triggers many illnesses, and even inhibits a normal healing process.

The type of stress caused by electromagnetic radiation is referred to as "electromagnetic stress."

What are the effects of electromagnetic pollution? How does electromagnetic stress affect people? We will address these questions in the next sections, and then go on to discuss crystals that may be of help.

The Symptoms of Electromagnetic Stress

The initial symptoms of electromagnetic stress frequently take the form of relatively non-specific disturbances in a person's general sense of well-being that cannot be pinned down to a specific cause, making the symptoms difficult to recognize.

A person might feel stressed, tired, or exhausted, suffer from circulatory problems and/or headaches, or often be ill. Their sleep patterns may be severely disrupted, they may develop an allergy or an existing allergy may be exacerbated. They may feel stressed mentally, and have feelings of anxiety and sadness, or depression. All these symptoms may equally be due to other causes, but exposure to electrosmog is often the underlying cause. Electromagnetic pollution may be a key contributory factor in serious illnesses such as cancer or autoimmune diseases, although these may not develop until years later, or they may develop due to multiple stress factors, including damaging environmental influences and psychological strain.

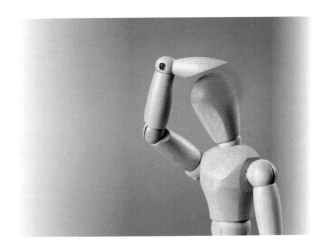

How Do the Symptoms Arise?

Electromagnetic pollution affects the human body by placing it under continual stress. In addition to other stress factors in modern daily life, stress from radiation (from electromagnetic pollution, for example) triggers a stress response in the body, with all the associated short- and long-term consequences. And if we are subjected to radiation on a continual basis, the response is stimulated repeatedly and the stress condition becomes chronic, leading first to constant overstimulation and finally to exhaustion within the body.

How and Why Does a Stress Response Occur?

Over the course of human evolution, the body has developed a program of reflexes in response to acute threats to its survival, preparing itself for a fight or flight response. Hormones are released that make the heart beat faster, and less blood is supplied to the skin and internal organs in favor of an increase in supply to the muscles and lungs. Blood sugar levels are raised to mobilize energy reserves and thought processes are superseded by automatic reflex actions. As a result, the mind's capacity to concentrate on a specific problem and think logically diminishes.

Normally these hormones are dissolved and eliminated after the acute threat has passed, and the body is then able to regain its natural balance. However, if the stress state is maintained through constant stimulation, grave long-term consequences can develop.

Long-term or permanent stress has become a serious problem in modern Western society and it has been an area of study for medical and psychological researchers for a number of years.

The Consequences of Permanent and Electromagnetic Stress

Stress Unbalances the Autonomic Nervous System

The autonomic nervous system (ANS) controls the body's "automatic" functions, those that take place without conscious effort. These include the heart function, circulation, and blood pressure, and the activities of other internal organs, along with muscle tension, the regulation of body temperature, and digestion.

Also controlled by the autonomic nervous system are our sense of balance, stress responses, the sleep-wake cycle, and other circadian rhythms. Consequently, the symptoms of a disturbance to any of the body processes controlled by the autonomic nervous system can be wide-ranging and each of us will react in our own way.

The symptoms of such a disturbance may include:

+ headaches

+ digestive problems

+ sleep disorders

+ circulatory problems, high or low blood pressure

+ heart rhythm disturbances

Stress and Metabolism, Increased Acidity in the Body, and Toxin Buildup

Metabolic processes cannot function properly in a body that is under continual stress. Persistent stress restricts blood flow to all the organs and tissues and impedes the normal working of the internal organs. The liver, stomach, intestines, pancreas, and kidneys are unable to function optimally, thus creating increased acidic metabolic waste products that cannot be eliminated effectively and are instead deposited in connective tissues. Over time this leads to acidosis, an excess of acid in the body.

Acidosis leads, for example, to headaches, joint and nerve pain, tiredness and a lack of energy, and muscle tension. It also encourages chronic inflammatory conditions.

Stress Adversely Affects the Proper Functioning of the Immune System

When the body is subjected to stress, the immune system's ability to protect it from disease and infection is reduced. If the stress continues unabated, for example as a result of persistent electromagnetic pollution, the outcome for the immune response can be highly detrimental. Chronic stress causes a reduction in the production of white blood cells (immune system cells that attack bacteria and viruses to fight off infection) and affects or suppresses the secretion of some hormones (chemical substances that control or regulate functions in the body such as digestion, growth, mood). This increases the likelihood of illness or indeed infections, which may heal more slowly or potentially become chronic themselves.

The Psychological Effects of Stress

The fact that stress makes us nervous and irritable is well known. However, the latest research has also proven a connection between stress and depression. In the field of building biology, it has been known for some time that electromagnetic stress may trigger depression, especially stress due to high frequency radiation (cell phones, radar, wifi, cordless telephones). It is also known that persistent stress, such as that caused by electromagnetic pollution, can have an influence on the body's production of hormones. The hormones serotonin and dopamine play particularly important roles in enhancing and stabilizing mood. When they are no longer produced in sufficient quantities, the result can be the triggering of depression.

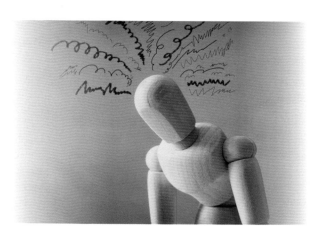

As we have seen, stress has far-reaching effects on our physical and psychological equilibrium. If persistent stress continues over a long period of time, serious illness such as cancer or autoimmune disease may be the result.

How to Deal with Electromagnetic Pollution

In order for the application of crystals to bring real and lasting relief, it is vital to reduce stress from radiation as much as possible; this is because crystals cannot eliminate radiation or even shield you from it, despite the many claims.

This is particularly relevant to all those devices that use modern radio technology: cell phones, cordless phones, devices using Bluetooth and wifi, along with electrical appliances and any electrical equipment that is kept in the bedroom.

Here are a few tips for reducing electrosmog within your own four walls at home:

✦ Use a cordless (portable) telephone that only transmits when you are using it; better still, use one where the handset/receiver is attached to the body of the phone with a cord.

✦ Don't use Bluetooth to connect to devices, and only activate wifi on your router or laptop/tablet when required.

✦ Don't use smart home apps, and if possible deactivate any transmitters in your household appliances and electrical devices (including plugs, LED lamps, switches, dimmers, heating thermostats, doorbells, cameras, robot vacuum cleaners, flower-watering systems, weather stations, air conditioning systems, thermometers, alarm systems, window and door sensors, cooking hobs, ovens, washing machines, refrigerators, coffee machines, televisions, hifi systems, loudspeakers, and radios).

✦ When buying a new device, check to see if it contains a transmitter and if so, ask if it can be deactivated.

✦ Don't use voice-activated assistants (such as Alexa, Siri).

✦ Smartphones:

– Deactivate wifi, Bluetooth, and mobile data when not in use.

– Install as few apps as possible and delete unused apps.

– Switch on flight mode whenever possible, **especially at night.**

– Use a headphone microphone or hands-free kit for calls.

✦ Take particular care to keep the room in which you sleep as free from radiation as possible. For example, smartphones and electrical devices that are switched on should not be left near your sleeping area. If you are aware that there is a significant amount of radiation coming into your bedroom from outside, or if you live in a residential area, with many people in close proximity to you, it may be necessary to give your bedroom special protection with radiation-shielding paint, or to protect your sleeping area with a canopy made from a radiation-shielding fabric.

You might also consider enlisting the help of a building biologist who specializes in electromagnetic pollution. They can measure the radiation stress levels in your home and suggest ways in which you can alleviate or reduce the problem.

Find out how to use crystals for relief in the pages that follow.

Using Crystals against Electromagnetic Pollution

In order to understand how crystals may help with stress that is caused by electromagnetic pollution, and yet equally to understand their limitations, we must first identify the differences between their various effects, both physical and energetic.

Physical Effects

An effect is physical when we can perceive it with one or more of our five senses, or when it can be measured using scientific equipment. Radiation from an electromagnetic field can be measured in specific units.* With cordless telephones, it is possible to measure exactly how much radiation a person is being exposed to when they stand at a certain distance from the phone's base station. If it is shielded with a suitable material, there is a clear difference in the measured values.

Energetic Effects

Some types of radiation are so subtle that they cannot be measured using conventional equipment. We generally call these types of radiation oscillations or vibrations.

This radiation is familiar to practitioners of homeopathy, those who use Bach Flower Remedies, and those who work with crystals. Its effect is generally referred to as energetic rather than physical.

Objective and Individual Effects

As a rule, physical phenomena can be perceived objectively. In other words, any measuring devices used will always register the same value, regardless of who is carrying out the test. The effects may be perceived subjectively, but they can still be verified by different people. After all, everyone will burn their fingers if they touch a hot stove!

* In µW/m2 (microwatts per meter squared, used for radio frequency [RF] radiation) or r V/m (volts per meter).

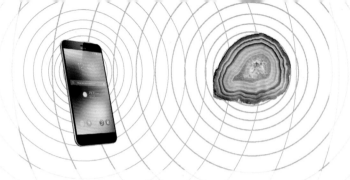

The subtler an oscillation or vibration, the more individual the perceived effect will be. One reason for this is that energetic oscillations mainly work through what is known as "resonance phenomena." The strength of a stimulus may be very low, but if the person being treated has within them structures (of a physical, emotional, mental nature, etc.) that resonate with the stimulus applied, the oscillation will be amplified and its effect will be dependent on the individual's own specific response.

The Correct Way to Deal with Electromagnetic Pollution

Since radiation and electromagnetic pollution initially have an effect on the human body that can be measured in a physical way, it follows that a physical approach should be our first port of call in protecting ourselves from electronic pollution. An appliance that emits radiation should be turned off, unless we have the means to protect* ourselves from it, just as we would turn off the burner on a cooker in order to protect our fingers, for example. No crystals or other energetic measures can protect us from burning our fingers. We can use them to treat a burn and alleviate pain, but they are not a preventative measure. The fact remains that if we do not remove our fingers from the burner on a stove, and/or do not switch if off, we will be burned. Even the most powerful of energetic healing measures will not change this.

* There are many different options for shielding against harmful electromagnetic fields, but please consult a professionally trained expert. (See addresses, page 79.)

How Crystals Can Protect Us

Crystals can never be a substitute for the physical actions that we can take to protect ourselves, nor can they replace measures that are based on the findings of building biology, or indeed taking a cautious approach to the whole question of radiation and modern technology at the outset.

Since they do not work in a physical but rather only in an energetic way, they cannot shield us from electromagnetic pollution, nor make it disappear. However, they are able to support both our physical and our energetic bodies in dealing with electromagnetic pollution's effects.

Crystals can only have an optimal effect when we remove as many as possible of the "coarse" physical stimuli (such as high radiation from some electronic devices) that interfere with or block our ability to react and resonate with our own energetic systems.

However, they can help us in the following ways:

✦ In coping with other inevitable stresses of modern life, while fortifying the body and the soul.

✦ In alleviating or healing the consequences of previous stress.

Crystals target those places in the body that have been particularly affected and damaged by stress from electromagnetic pollution. A number of crystals are traditionally used to deal with the effects of this form of pollution, and we discuss each separately.

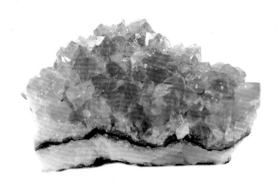

Notes on the descriptions of the effects of crystals

Many of the crystals described can be used in a number of areas relating to electromagnetic pollution and could therefore feature in more than one section, but we describe them in detail in the section that covers their main effects. At the end of every section you will find the *Additional Crystals* listing, which details crystals that are described in another section but are still effective for the subject matter being discussed. The page number given after each crystal refers to where you can find its detailed description. Relevant keywords for each crystal are featured in brackets for your reference.

For example, garnet in the *Regeneration* section is shown as:
Garnet: Page 49 (→ Immune System, Metabolism).

Classic Electromagnetic Pollution Crystals

Certain crystals are frequently associated with treating electronic pollution. Generally speaking, they are used for any type of disturbance, and often no distinction is made between radiation from the Earth ("geopathic stress") and physical radiation from electromagnetic radiation. There is a great deal of false information in circulation (not to mention many persistent myths), along with plenty of misunderstandings about their application.

Clear Quartz

At one time clear quartz was believed to be effective against electromagnetic radiation. It was thought to work by attracting the radiation and drawing it away and was used to protect against radiation from monitor screens. The crystals would be attached to the monitors, with their tips pointing away from the user. Clear quartz can indeed draw energy from its base toward its tip and this property of gathering or "bundling" energy and conducting it away through the tip is used in energetic treatments in particular.

Light is also gathered and conducted within clear quartz. However, unfortunately the same does not apply to other types of radiation, including electrical and electromagnetic radiation as emitted by computer monitor screens and other appliances. Clear quartz cannot conduct the radiation away and in addition, if it is badly positioned, clear quartz may even exacerbate the problem.

Clear quartz is inherently neutral and is therefore able to absorb information, store it, and pass it on. This means that in a worst-case scenario, a piece of clear quartz crystal placed on a "disturbance," for example, will even amplify negative oscillations and spread them throughout an entire room. These waves will radiate from both its tip and its edges. The level of physical radiation, which can be measured technically, will not change due to the crystal—the amount of radiation will not increase or decrease, so nothing really changes in that respect. The energetic information coming from the disturbance can, however, become amplified under certain conditions and may negatively affect the climate of the whole room. **Clear quartz should therefore never be placed on any points of disturbance, no matter what type, and the position chosen for placing the crystal should be tested with suitable means beforehand.** If you wish to influence the climate of a room in a beneficial way, place a clear quartz crystal in a positive zone of the room so that it will radiate the zone's positive qualities.

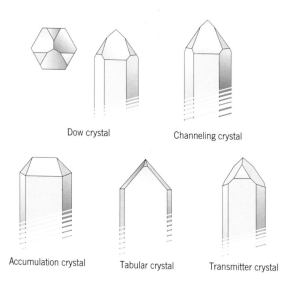

Dow crystal

Channeling crystal

Accumulation crystal

Tabular crystal

Transmitter crystal

A crystal may also be carried in the hand as a comforting object, or worn on the body, perhaps as a pendant. Since electromagnetic stress draws energy from the body, the properties of clear quartz may have a very positive effect. As a neutral energy supplier, it can strengthen the body and spirit and make you less susceptible to negative external influences. It improves perception, brings clarity, and makes you generally more aware on a conscious level. You may, therefore, be better able to recognize disturbances in your surroundings and have the means for removing them more quickly, before they have the capacity to cause greater damage.

The use of special clear quartz crystals may also be very helpful: **Dow crystal** balances out a lack or excess of energy in the body and strengthens self-organizing abilities. **Faden** quartz can strengthen the body's self-healing properties. **Channeling crystals** improve the body's awareness and recognition of its own needs. Thanks to their property of building up or collecting, **accumulation crystals** help to gather energy and to better manage the body's energy reserves. They help to conduct away excess energy and clear a room's atmosphere. **Tabular crystals** amplify all the body's energies and **transmitter crystals** improve a person's communication with their body.

Clear quartz is also excellent for combining in an application with other crystals, since it amplifies their strength.

Rose Quartz

Rose quartz is another well-known crystal that is often used for counteracting interference. As a general rule, no distinction is made between technical radiation and geopathic stress radiation from the Earth in terms of the application of rose quartz. As a result, it is used both for electromagnetic stress and for stress from an Earth source, such as water veins and similar phenomena. Placing an unworked rose quartz crystal beside or under the bed, or on an electrical device, is often recommended in order to "earth" its radiation.

However, in this context the term "earthing" is a little misleading. It is possible to earth electrical and electromagnetic fields as a shielding measure, but a crystal can never accomplish this from a physical perspective. Even on an energetic level, the argument for using a crystal in an earthing capacity is tenuous at best.

Aside from that, rose quartz is a great crystal. When analyzed with a dowsing rod or pendulum, you can see that it emits almost exclusively positive oscillations. In principle, this means that it can influence the climate of a room in a positive manner. Hence, working energetically, it can create a certain balance for disturbances that otherwise cannot be removed. Thanks to this effect, it can make interfering radiation more tolerable for a period of time, on both a mental and spiritual level.

However, as with other crystals, the problem is that its influence is restricted and will eventually be completely exhausted. Depending on the strength and the type of radiation, it will only work for a number of hours or days, after which time the opposite effect occurs. This means that in order to use a crystal's potential effectively and sensibly, you must check its effect at least on a daily basis and then regularly cleanse and recharge the crystal (see page 73). Here too, the following applies: the less intense the radiation, the longer the crystal will retain its positive effect.

The truth is that adopting measures to carry out effective energetic suppression is usually at least as time-consuming as changing around your sleeping location or taking an approach based on physical building biology. In addition, the positive energetic effect of rose quartz can only work properly over longer periods if the physical causes of the radiation have been reduced as much as possible. Rose quartz should therefore only be employed to reduce radiation in combination with building biology, when its harmonizing property will unfold to its full potential.

This crystal also has the effect of making you feel awake. So, if you have trouble getting to sleep or sleeping through the night, don't place rose quartz near your bed.

Finally, rose quartz also improves sensitivity; it reinforces empathy and the ability to love and be helpful. It also harmonizes the heart rhythm and strengthens the heart.

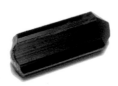

Black Tourmaline (Schorl)
Tourmaline Quartz (Schorl in Quartz)

Black tourmaline is a classic protection crystal. It shields from external influences, mainly energetic. Practitioners often recommend placing it between yourself and the source of radiation, such as a computer monitor screen. However, as with all other crystals, it cannot shield you physically, so we recommend wearing it on the body where its positive energetic properties may take effect more successfully. If you have exhausted all the possibilities for protection based on building biology, black tourmaline may also help to make any remaining radiation more tolerable by dissolving blockages in the flow of energy.

For example, it can be extremely effective when traveling and you find it is simply not possible to avoid being in a room that is subject to high levels of radiation. In such instances, using black tourmaline, perhaps in a necklace, may help to compensate for the effects of radiation for a limited amount of time.

All types of tourmaline have an essentially stimulating effect on the body's energy flow, with black tourmaline being the most useful in this respect. It also improves communication across the various levels of function in the human body, connecting spirit, soul, mind, and body in a single harmonious whole. What better prerequisite is there for a healthy and happy life?

One of the main problems with electromagnetic stress is that the radiation it emits greatly affects the communication processes within the body. In order for the human body to function in all its complexity, its cells, organs, and organ systems need to be able to exchange information on their activities on a continuous basis so that these activities can be coordinated. In this context, radiation constitutes a significant disturbance, preventing the optimal exchange of information. This, in turn, causes control disruptions, energetic blockages, and finally illness.

Black tourmaline helps to reestablish energy flow and the healthy exchange of information, and it can even help to prevent large disruptions to energy flow.

The color black is, in itself, indicative of the setting of boundaries. Its other characteristics also make it suitable for combating the effects of electromagnetic stress. Tourmaline alleviates stress, is helpful in cases of muscle tension and pain, and encourages sleep.

Tourmaline quartz consists of fine, needle-shaped inclusions of tourmaline embedded in clear quartz. In principle, it works in the same way as black tourmaline.

Tourmaline quartz dissolves stress, tension, and resistance. It has an enlivening and activating effect—more so even than black tourmaline—and thus helps to find a balance between tension and relaxation. The body is therefore able to react to external influences appropriately and in the best possible way, and to counterbalance any disturbances.

Smoky Quartz/Morion

Smoky quartz is formed when quartz is subjected to natural radioactive radiation from the surrounding rock. It increases resistance to radiation and alleviates radiation damage. It has a very strong relaxing effect and is regarded as a classic anti-stress crystal.

Electromagnetic pollution in particular causes a constant stress reaction in the body, a kind of permanent state of unease or anxiety that persists until the body's energy reserves are exhausted. The symptoms include tension and headaches, restlessness, irritability, sleep disturbances, nervousness, and digestive problems. The usual outcome is chronic exhaustion and a reduced immune response, opening the door to further disease.

In such cases, smoky quartz may help to dissolve any tension. It heightens our ability to withstand stress and strengthens our nerves so that we become less susceptible to external influences.

Smoky quartz is excellent for dealing with the acute symptoms of radiation stress. However, in the long term it cannot compensate for severe stress. Instead, the causes of the stress need to be addressed so that it can be reduced to a level where the body can manage without the help of the crystal. Smoky quartz should be warn directly on the body for extended periods of time. It can also be worn on painful or tense points on the body. For relaxation, use two large tumbled crystals or hold a crystal in each hand.

Morion is a special, dark (almost black) smoky quartz that has been exposed to particularly strong radiation. As a result, it is very effective against radiation influence.

Tektite

Tektite is formed when a large meteorite hits the Earth. Both the meteorite and the rock that it strikes here on Earth evaporate on impact. Splashes of molten matter are flung out in the explosion and solidify in the air.

Tektite encourages us to realize that we are spiritual beings and strengthens our empathetic and clairvoyant abilities. It brings spontaneity, impulsiveness, and new ideas, and it frees us from anxiety and attachment to material things.

Tektite appears to have a very positive influence on stress caused by electromagnetic pollution, especially the kind caused by high frequency radiation (cell phones, cordless telephones, and so on). Kinesiological tests show that the body appears to react less strongly to a cell phone conversation if a piece of tektite is being carried at the time. It would seem, therefore, that tektite can improve our ability to cope with and help compensate for this radiation, at least for a short time. However, that does not mean that the radiation is harmless or does not leach energy from the body. Even armed with a tektite crystal, in the long run frequent exposure to radiation stress will lead to severe depletion of the body's energy reserves. Tektite can occasionally be used to cope with unavoidable stress in certain circumstances, but prevention is the preferred option—it's always best to simply avoid unnecessary exposure to damaging radiation whenever possible.

As a general rule, tektite can assist with all strong physical, spiritual, and mental stress, in order to help us to be able to "switch off" when necessary. So when stress is severe, we can also use it to create some space, giving ourselves time to take action. This will not be effective in the long term, however. We still need to identify and remove the causes of the stress.

On a physical level, tektite crystal encourages healing. It does so by prompting awareness of the causes of an illness. It is especially helpful in the case of infectious diseases.

Tip: When the Crystal Healing Association tested tektite, it found that the crystal may actually activate latent or potential diseases. In the end, this may be viewed as part of the healing process, but it may also be rather unpleasant if you aren't expecting it!

Tektite may help those who find it difficult to get to sleep or whose sleep is disturbed during the night. Try drinking tektite crystal water before going to sleep and placing a tektite crystal under your pillow.

The Immune System

Another key aspect of electromagnetic pollution is its effects on the body's immune system. It has been proven that this form of pollution weakens the immune defenses and even opens the door to infections and severe illness.

The functioning of the immune system is extremely complex and various of its aspects play a part in our physical, mental, and spiritual health. This is why we have not dealt with it in a separate section—the issues and solutions described in the sections that follow provide the foundation for a healthy and properly functioning immune system.

Many crystals are capable of fortifying the immune system. As a rule, they do so by assisting in one of the aspects described on the following pages.

Protection and Boundary Setting

The ability to create proper boundaries in life plays an essential role in maintaining good health and ensuring well-being. The better we are at setting boundaries, the better we will be protected from outside influences. This can be seen most easily on a physical level. The skin and the mucus membranes act as a barrier, together preventing foreign substances from entering the body. If the skin is damaged or the mucus membranes can no longer fulfill their function correctly, harmful organisms can invade the body and cause disease. But protecting ourselves from external influences on a mental and spiritual level, too, is equally essential for good health. The two are closely connected. Experience shows that people who are able to establish boundaries in their emotional and spiritual lives usually have a strong immune system and are not easily unbalanced by external influences. Thus, as a rule, they also react with less sensitivity to electromagnetic pollution.

The following pages feature descriptions of crystals that encourage positive boundary setting on a physical, mental, and spiritual level. Most also strengthen the immune system.

Agate

There are a number of different types of agate, with each affecting a specific area of the body, depending on their signature or marking. Banded agates are particularly suitable for protecting against electromagnetic pollution. They balance the aura and the energetic bodies, and ensure that a strong, protective, enveloping shield is created on the energetic plane.

Agate encourages spiritualization, focus, concentration, and the ability to deal with our life experiences with awareness. In this way, agate allows us to grow and mature spiritually, leading to inner stability and a sound sense of reality. It dissolves internal tension and brings safety, security, and protection, helping us to be more stable in the face of external influences. On a general level, it encourages a logical, pragmatic, and well-grounded attitude to life.

Thunder Eggs

Also called star agates or amulet stones, they stimulate the liver (detoxification) and the immune system. In addition, they stabilize our physical and mental constitution.

Mica

All minerals in the mica group produce good protective crystals, as do other types of rock containing large proportions of mica. They help with boundary setting and support a person's sense of their own identity and autonomy. They also have a detoxifying effect.

The following crystals containing mica are particularly interesting in connection with the symptoms of electromagnetic stress:

Biotite

Biotite lens is considered a classic protective crystal in Portugal, where it originates. Biotite strengthens our resolve to fulfill our own potential; it helps to free us from being "pigeonholed" by others and from their demands. It motivates us to achieve our own ideas and to make decisions. On a physical level, it works as a detoxifying crystal, as do all the crystals containing mica; it helps to balance an excess of acidity and is effective for rheumatism, gout, and sciatica.

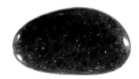

Lepidolite (Mica containing lithium)

Lepidolite protects from external influences and helps with boundary setting. It encourages autonomy and self-discipline. Lepidolite can be applied to alleviate painful conditions that may arise in connection with electromagnetic stress, such as neuralgia (nerve) pain, including sciatica, and pain from joint problems.

In addition, it has a detoxifying effect, balancing an excess of acid in the body and stimulating the cleansing processes of the skin and the connective tissues.

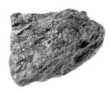

Fuchsite

Fuchsite is a type of mica that contains chromium. It helps facilitate boundary setting, while also remaining alert and attentive to the external world. It allows us to view our worries from a distance, but without denying that they exist. Fuchsite encourages creative problem-solving and keeps the spirit and body flexible. Especially important in terms of electromagnetic stress, fuchsite fortifies the immune system and encourages detoxification. It alleviates the sudden onset of inflammations, and helps the body to deal with allergies and other conditions that produce eruptions on the skin accompanied by itching and scaliness.

Fuchsite with ruby is particularly interesting in connection with electromagnetic pollution, as the protective and detoxifying effects of the fuchsite merge with the vitalizing and fortifying powers of the ruby (see also Ruby, page 50).

Aventurine

Aventurine contains both quartz and fuchsite, and so is classed with those crystals that contain mica. You will find it described in detail in the *Harmonization and Balance* section.

Heliotrope

Heliotrope is a green chalcedony with inclusions of yellow and red jasper. It helps us to set boundaries and protect ourselves from, and keep at bay, unwanted external influences. It promotes flexibility and the ability to adapt without compromising our own point of view. It also brings strength when we feel exhausted or tired, while at the same time relieving irritability and nervousness.

On a physical level, heliotrope is also one of the most effective crystals for fortifying the immune system, especially in those suffering from an acute infection. It stimulates the flow of lymph and the metabolism, and detoxifies and neutralizes an excess of acid.

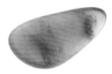

Serpentine

Serpentine is another classic protective crystal. Thanks to its layered structure, it strengthens the ability to set boundaries. On a physical level it relieves pain from cramp and helps to combat an excess of acid in the body. It also helps to balance mood swings, along with promoting inner peace.

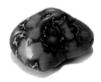

Turquoise

Turquoise is one of the best known protective crystals. It makes us less sensitive to external influences by strengthening our sense of identity and mobilizing our energy reserves. It makes us conscious of being in control of our life and destiny, and helps us to find the strength and the courage to bring about change, should that become necessary. It helps us to take our life into our own hands and control it from a place of personal power. Turquoise also balances mood swings. Especially useful in terms of electromagnetic stress, turquoise has a pain-relieving effect and dissolves cramp, soothes inflammations, detoxifies, and dissolves acidification.

Additional crystals for protection and boundary setting:

Jade (Jadeite/Nephrite) Page 58 (→ Metabolism, Elimination)

Strengthening Life Energy: Power and Vitality

Stress from electromagnetic pollution not only drains our strength physically, but also, ultimately, mentally and spiritually, too. The following crystals may help to mobilize energy reserves for a time, but without simultaneously amplifying or stimulating the stress too much. They bring vitality and the energy to deal with stressful situations more easily.

Applying these crystals makes sense, even in situations where electromagnetic stress has been present for a significant amount of time, and where long-term stress has led to serious illness or extensive physical and mental exhaustion.

Garnet

Garnet has a broad regenerating quality and strengthens resistance. It fortifies resolve and in times of crisis brings stamina and endurance, courage and trust. It helps us to glimpse the light at the end of the tunnel, and, when it seems as though none of our actions are taking effect, it helps us to overcome our doubts and do whatever is necessary.

When severe stress from electromagnetic pollution has been present for some time, many people reach a point where they feel they can no longer carry on, especially if the stress has not been recognized and doctors can find no cause for what are often severe symptoms.

Many patients for whom all treatment options have failed find themselves categorized as having a complaint that is "all in the mind," and subsequently lose all hope of improvement or cure. In such instances, garnet may bring renewed hope and confidence. It may help the patient find their own path to recovery and overcome external resistance.

Above all, garnet strengthens the body's powers of regeneration and removes energetic blockages. In addition, it stimulates the metabolism and improves the consistency of the body's fluids. It stabilizes the blood circulation, fortifies the immune system, and accelerates the healing of internal and external injuries (wounds).

Ruby

Ruby brings strength and *joie de vivre*, vitality and dynamism, but without overstimulating us into hyperactivity. It improves self-confidence, efficiency, and productivity. It helps when we are feeling discouraged and exhausted, which may also be the consequences of long-term stress, such as from electromagnetic pollution. Ruby may also stimulate new ideas and a readiness to take action in those who have tried many ways to heal their suffering and have subsequently lost hope.

On a physical level, ruby stimulates the spleen, the adrenal glands, and the circulation. It supports the immune system and helps to combat infectious diseases. It activates the entire metabolism and may also help the body to recover its ability to respond, so that other natural healing measures can prove effective once more.

Red Jasper

Red jasper promotes dynamism and activity, but without the impulsiveness sometimes associated with ruby.

It stimulates the circulation and the body's energy flow. Jasper encourages willpower, courage, and a readiness to face conflict, making it easier to initiate necessary changes and to persevere with any therapy that may be already underway.

Hematite

Hematite lends strength, vitality, and liveliness. It is effective almost exclusively on the physical level. It improves the gut's ability to absorb iron and supports the formation of red blood cells, thereby improving the overall supply of oxygen to the entire body.

Tiger Iron

Tiger iron consists of a number of alternating layers (bands) of tiger eye, jasper, and hematite, and combines the positive qualities of all three crystals. It heightens vitality, as well as fortifying strength, dynamism, and endurance. It is therefore of help when the body lacks iron (anemia), and feels tired and exhausted. It encourages the absorption of iron, the formation of red blood cells, and the supply of oxygen to the body. Tiger iron has a rapid effect and can therefore be applied when energy reserves are severely depleted.

Mookaite

Mookaite is a colorful variety of chert, and a mixture of jasper and opal. Indigenous Australians still use it as an energizing healing stone.

Mookaite brings vitality and dynamism, together with internal focus, peace, and balance. It also promotes liveliness, which is realized in harmonious activity rather than in simply draining the body's resources. It helps us to decide how much we need to contribute in a given situation, and encourages us to only do as much as is needed and is good for us. In this way, we can enjoy realizing our projects and ideas.

Mookaite's key physical effect is cleansing the blood in the liver and spleen. It reinforces the body's vitality and the immune system. It also helps to stabilize health in the long term. Like jasper, mookaite boosts vitality and the strength of the whole body. It should be worn for an extended period of time in order for it to develop its full effect.

Strengthening the Center: Stability

Stressful situations are best handled when we are fully aware of our own resources and can face a situation with internal calm and focus. The crystals- described in the following section strengthen our "center" and Earth connectedness. They encourage a relaxed attitude, and both stability, and endurance, and in so doing provide the optimal basis for dealing with environmental stresses.

Dendritic Agate (Tree Agate)

Dendritic agate promotes persistence, security, and stability, as well as endurance, even in unpleasant situations, and makes us aware of our own strength and resources. It therefore helps us to take on and deal with challenges. It encourages vitality in the body and good, stable health. Dendritic agate fortifies resistance and the immune system, and also helps with susceptibility to infection. It should be worn for an extended period of time in order for its effect to fully unfold.

Brown and Yellow Jasper

Brown and yellow jasper mainly support endurance and stamina. They encourage focus and impart inner calm, while fortifying the immune system in the long term. They are especially helpful with diseases of the gut and the digestive organs.

Petrified Wood

Petrified wood encourages a strong and robust sense of reality and has a grounding effect.

It helps to center and calm our focus, so that energy is released over the long term without exhausting the body's reserves. It helps us to become aware of the signals that our body sends us and to listen and respond to them, and it brings a sense of well-being and an ability to take pleasure in the simple things in life.

On a physical level, petrified wood stabilizes good health and brings energy, as well as aiding recovery. It activates the metabolism and calms the nerves, and is therefore very beneficial when we feel "wound up," restless, and nervous, symptoms that often arise when the body has been subjected to electromagnetic stress.

Opalized Petrified Wood (where the petrified wood has developed an opalescent sheen or is composed of opal) also encourages detoxification and elimination.

Additional crystals for stability:
Agate: Page 43 (→ Immune System)
Star Agate: Page 44 (→ Immune System, Detoxification)
Mookaite: Page 52 (→ Immune System)
Ocean Jasper: Page 55 (→ Immune System, Detoxification)

Regeneration

The stress caused by electromagnetic pollution can burden us to such an extent that we reach the limits of our physical and mental abilities to withstand that stress, and it may, in the long term, even trigger serious illnesses. This is particularly the case when our health is affected over the long term and the causes are recognized late or sometimes even not at all. This can often lead to exhaustion and the feeling that there is no way out. Thankfully, some crystals can help to bolster our courage and to stimulate the body's powers of regeneration, on a physical and mental level.

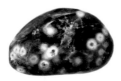

Ocean Jasper

Strictly speaking, ocean jasper is not a jasper at all, but rather a rhyolite containing quartz, which means it is classed as a volcanic crystal. It is also known as ocean agate.

Ocean jasper encourages a positive outlook on life and helps us to withstand stress and remain calm through self-acceptance. It also encourages healthy sleep. Physically, it strengthens the immune system and promotes detoxification, as well as being of assistance in cases of flu, stubborn colds, cysts, and tumors. As a result, it is also beneficial in alleviating the consequences of electromagnetic stress.

Epidote

Epidote helps us to recognize our situation and makes us conscious of the reality around us. It encourages change in a measured way and having the patience required to translate our wishes and goals into reality with pragmatism. It also encourages recuperation and regeneration on all levels—physical, mental, and spiritual. It helps to strengthen our ability to be productive and efficient, reinforces the constitution, and with this same property of building up and fortifying, it supports healing. Epidote can therefore help to stabilize the immune system and stimulate liver function and the digestive processes.

It can also be successfully applied to encourage regeneration after a severe cold or a bout of serious stress. It helps us to be patient enough to allow recuperation and recovery to take place, enabling us to evaluate realistically what is possible and what would place too many demands on the body and therefore trigger a relapse.

Zoisite

Zoisite helps us to overcome destructive mental attitudes and the feeling that we cannot alter our future. It promotes creativity and the ability to take our lives into our own hands. It encourages us to develop our goals and new ideas, and helps to free us from a tendency to be too accommodating in respect of others or to allow our lives to be governed by external factors.

On a physical level, zoisite stimulates cell renewal and the regeneration of the entire body. It also promotes recuperation after great stress and serious illness, as well as assisting with detoxification and the neutralization of too much acid in the body. It inhibits inflammations and strengthens the immune system.

Zoisite is also available in the form of **zoisite with ruby**. The crystals complement each other's effects very well, especially when they are applied for issues that are a result of electromagnetic pollution.

Zoisite takes effect slowly and should therefore be worn for longer periods of time in direct contact with skin.

Additional crystals for regeneration:
Garnet: Page 49 (→ Immune System, Metabolism)
Brown Tourmaline (Dravite): Page 60 (→ Metabolism, Autonomic Nervous System)
Emerald: Page 68 (→ Metabolism, Immune System, Harmonization and Balance)

Harmonization and Balance

Electromagnetic stress is a strong interference impulse that causes imbalance in both the body and the mind. It severely disrupts the body's natural physical regulatory systems, which in the long term also affects our emotional balance, too.

Electromagnetic stress targets conditions that are acute—for example, instances where the immune system has overreacted, perhaps resulting in an allergic reaction, an autoimmune illness, or even a weakening of the immune system itself. Similarly, it may target the over- or underproduction of hormones, conditions that are frequently connected with severe mood swings, among other issues. The crystals featured in the following pages have been selected for their balancing effects and their properties of helping to calm down and harmonize any physical and mental overreactions.

Jade (Jadeite/Nephrite)

The term jade is used to describe two very different minerals with similar effects: jadeite and nephrite. Jadeite is extremely rare, while most crystals described as jade are usually nephrite.

Jade contains different mineral substances, some of which have a stimulating and some a calming effect. Hence, jade brings the balance that we need in life, spurring us into action when we are feeling lethargic and calming us in times of stress or irritability. In the long term, it promotes stability and inner balance, along with a sense of proportion and measure in all things. At the same time, jade also makes us mentally active and proactive. It helps to strengthen our sense of our own identity, as well as being a classic protective crystal against harmful external influences.

On a physical level, jade stimulates kidney function and so balances the levels of water, salts, and acid/alkaline fluids in the body. It also stimulates the nervous system and regulates the function of the adrenal glands. It therefore has a balancing effect on the production of the stress hormones adrenaline and noradrenaline, which place the body in a state of readiness in an emergency (the fight or flight response). An increased release of these hormones often plays an important role in the reaction to electromagnetic pollution. In such cases, jade is able to provide balance and restore the body's ability to react, so that it is better able to deal with illness and therapy blockages.

 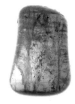 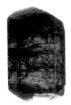

Tourmaline

Tourmaline is one of the most diverse crystals in the mineral kingdom as it occurs in many different colors. Depending on its color, it has a wide range of healing effects, multicolored tourmaline is particularly appropriate for issues that concern balance and harmony. It helps bring the spirit, psyche, intellect, and body together into a harmonious whole. It helps us to be more open and flexible, stimulates the energy flow in the meridians, and helps to dissolve blockages. On a physical level, it assists in fortifying where there is weakness. It harmonizes the nerves, metabolism, hormonal glands, and immune system. If there is no multicoloured tourmaline to hand, a combination (in a mix that feels right to you) of the following single colors is particularly recommended:

Rubellite (red tourmaline) improves energy flow and the conductivity of the nerves. It strengthens the functions of the sexual organs, and encouraging a good blood supply and blood cleansing in the spleen and liver. **Verdelite (green tourmaline)** fortifies the heart and has a detoxifying effect. It also supports elimination. **Dravite (brown-yellow tourmaline)** stimulates the regenerative powers of the body's cells, tissues, and organs.

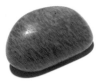

Amazonite

On a physical level, amazonite regulates metabolic problems, eases pain from cramp, and has a general relaxing effect. It strengthens the nerves and harmonizes the autonomic nervous system and the internal organs. Mentally and spiritually, amazonite balances mood swings. It has a calming effect and promotes trust. It helps us to get rid of the sense of being a victim of a cruel fate, at the same time encouraging us to take back control of our lives.

Aventurine

Aventurine is a quartz with a glistening, green appearance that is due to the inclusion of fuchsite. It combines the best effects of quartz (see clear quartz, page 46) and fuchsite.

Aventurine has repeatedly proven effective in helping to prevent and heal damage from radiation. It promotes resistance to radiation stress and rapidly alleviates its unpleasant side effects, such as headaches or other types of pain, nervous complaints, autonomic nervous system disorders, and skin irritations.

It is beneficial in cases of nervousness, stress, and sleep disorders, and relaxes the body and mind. It also frees us from external influences and demands. Aventurine is therefore highly effective in dealing with the burdens that electromagnetic pollution places on us, both mentally and physically, the constant stress of which may often lead to the symptoms just mentioned. It is particularly helpful for people who place great demands upon and tend to expect too much of themselves. It also helps us to "switch off" if we are worrying too much about a potential stress and its consequences.

Additional crystals for harmonization and balance:
Serpentine: Page 47 (→ Metabolism)
Emerald: Page 68 (→ Metabolism, Immune System, Regeneration)
Rose Quartz: Page 36 (a classic electromagnetic pollution crystal)
Sunstone: Page 62
Amber: Page 63

Strengthening the Autonomic Nervous System

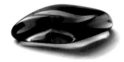

Ametrine

Ametrine is a combination of amethyst and citrine. It promotes *joie de vivre*, creativity, and optimism, and the general sense of being in control of our lives. On a mental level, it encourages harmony and emotional well-being, which is also helpful in stressful situations. On a physical level, it has a cleansing effect and activates the cellular metabolism, which is frequently severely disrupted by electromagnetic stress. This crystal also strengthens the autonomic nervous system and harmonizes the interaction between the internal organs, promoting harmony and vitality in the whole body.

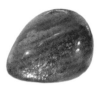

Sunstone

Sunstone activates the body's healing powers. It stimulates the autonomic nervous system and harmonizes the interaction between the organs. Mentally and spiritually, sunstone lends *joie de vivre* and optimism. It lightens the mood and has antidepressant properties. It also increases our sense of self-worth and self-confidence.

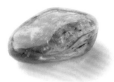

Amber

Amber brings happiness and trust, promoting a carefree, sunny disposition and strengthening our belief in ourselves. In this way we can feel better centered and able to react flexibly to external conditions without losing our centeredness. Physically, amber assists with issues concerning the joints and fortifies the mucus membranes. It stimulates wound healing, is beneficial in the case of stomach, spleen, and kidney complaints, and has a positive effect on the liver and gall bladder.

Additional crystals for fortifying the autonomic nervous system:
Amazonite: Page 60 (→ Metabolism)
Tourmaline: Page 59 (→ Metabolism)

Metabolism and Detoxification

Metabolism is the collective term for the absorption, transportation, and chemical transformation of substances in an organism and the release of metabolic products into the environment. The processes involved include, for example, respiration, digestion, and many others in which one substance is transformed into another. The functioning of these processes is very complex and can easily be disturbed through stress from electromagnetic pollution. The result is an increase in the amount of waste products from incomplete or even compromised transformation processes, such as free radicals and damaging acids. These waste products are transported around the body by the blood cells, but primarily by the white lymph fluid. The lymph fluid is located in the spaces between the cells in the so-called connective tissue and is transported via the lymph channels to the body's excretory organs. Metabolic end products are also temporarily stored in the connective tissue and are absorbed by the lymph.

However, if too many waste products are stored they clog up the connective tissues, and the lymph can no longer eliminate them. The tissues become congested with toxic waste, upsetting the pH balance of the entire body. Healthy functioning metabolic and lymphatic systems are vital for maintaining good health.

As already mentioned, electromagnetic stress may significantly disturb the metabolic processes and impair the correct functioning of the lymphatic system.

Electromagnetic pollution increases acidity in the tissues and can therefore be accompanied by a number of consequences that are all too familiar: pain, tension, chronic inflammations, a weakening of the immune system, fatigue, hair loss, osteoporosis, and the encouraging of carcinogenic conditions, among others.

The following crystals may be useful in addressing these problems:

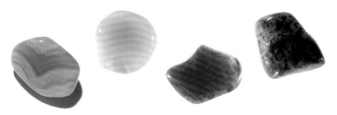

Chalcedony Family

As a general rule, chalcedony crystals bring lightness and openness, and the ability to make friends easily, along with an improved ability to communicate with others.

Blue chalcedony, the best known representative of the chalcedony family, encourages flexibility, helps us to deal with inner resistance, and promotes inner calm.

On a physical level, blue chalcedony and banded chalcedony stimulate the flow of bodily fluids, especially lymph, and so help to reduce water retention in the tissues (edemas), eliminate metabolic waste products, and strengthen the immune system. **Pink chalcedony** may also be useful when the heart function needs strengthening, while **red chalcedony** has a stimulating effect on the circulation when blood pressure is low.

Copper chalcedony also stimulates the metabolism of copper and the detoxification processes of the liver.

Dendritic Agate

Dendritic (tree) agate has a detoxifying effect and encourages the elimination of metabolic waste products from the tissues.

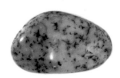

Opalite

Opalite encourages sociability and contact with our surroundings and other people. On a physical level, it fortifies the mucus membranes.

Opalite also stimulates the function of the lungs, encourages the absorption of oxygen, and helps to combat the symptoms of a tenacious common cold that is hard to shake off and the effects on the body of smoking. It encourages the elimination of waste products, as well as detoxification and digestive processes, while also cleansing the connective tissues, intestines, and mucus membranes.

Additional crystals for the metabolism and elimination processes:

Turquoise: Page 48 (→ Detoxification)

Heliotrope: Page 47 (→ Immune System, Power and Vitality, Detoxification)

Serpentine: Page 47 (→ Harmonization and Balance)

Garnet: Page 49 (→ Immune System)

Zoisite: Page 56 (→ Immune System, Detoxification)

Zoisite with ruby: Page 57 (→ Immune System, Detoxification, Power and Vitality)

Ametrine: Page 62 (→ Harmonization and Balance, Detoxification)

Colored Tourmaline: Page 59 (→ Immune System, Autonomic Nervous System)

Amazonite: Page 60 (→ Autonomic Nervous System)

Detoxification and Elimination

Multiple stresses on the body due to exposure to other toxic substances can produce an increased sensitivity to electromagnetic pollution, for example, exposure to heavy metals from the environment or from amalgam tooth fillings. Detoxifying the body generally results in a noticeable decrease in the symptoms caused by stress and the crystals described in the following pages can help to set this process in motion. We have chosen those crystals that tend to have a gentle effect, one that stabilizes us physically and mentally and will not usually produce a severe reaction to the detoxification process. That said, take care if you are already suffering from serious illness or if you know you have been exposed to toxins at a high level. Existing symptoms may worsen drastically during detoxification, or even cause the symptoms of previous illnesses to return. In such cases, consult a natural medicine practitioner or physician if you wish to apply these crystals.

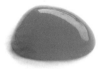

Chrysoprase

Chrysoprase belongs to the chalcedony family. It therefore improves the flow of the bodily fluids, especially lymph, and encourages the elimination of waste products.

Through its inclusion of nickel, which also gives it its apple-green coloring, chrysoprase has a strong detoxifying effect. It can even stimulate the elimination of heavy metals and other substances that do not dissolve easily. This crystal is also excellent for supporting the liver. Chrysoprase helps us to deal with illnesses that are due to poisoning, and it is also useful against allergies, skin disease, and rheumatism.

On a mental and spiritual level, chrysoprase has a cleansing and dissolving effect. It helps us to work through stressful experiences, to overcome any negative feelings, and to free ourselves from unhelpful thoughts, directing our attention toward a positive outcome. It promotes feelings of trust and security. It also helps us to "sort ourselves out," and to experience an all-embracing feeling of the recognition of our place in the world and the deep trust that comes from being part of a greater whole, to which we can contribute in ways that are in keeping with ourselves and our capabilities.

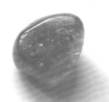

Green Garnet

The green varieties of garnet, tsavorite, and uvarovite are particularly good at stimulating detoxification, and also have an anti-inflammatory effect. Tsavorite, in particular, also brings renewed strength in difficult times and helps us to face problems and overcome difficulties.

For its mental and spiritual effects, see garnet in the *Strengthing Life Energy* section.

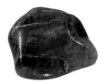

Emerald

Emerald brings alertness, clarity, and farsightedness, and encourages a sense of beauty, esthetics, harmony, and justice. It helps us to find a new direction when crises occur in our lives and supports us in identifying goals and finding meaning.

Emerald accelerates spiritual growth and strengthens the ability to regenerate and rejuvenate. It is particularly effective for inflammations of the upper respiratory tract and nasal sinus cavities. It stimulates liver function, encourages detoxification and de-acidification, and helps us to deal with typical disorders due to high levels of acid in the body, such as rheumatism or gout. It also assists with alleviating pain and strengthens the immune system.

Additional crystals for detoxification and elimination:

Turquoise: Page 48 (→ Metabolism)

Mica: Page 44

Lepidolite: Page 45 (→ Metabolism and Detoxification)

Fuchsite: Page 46 (→ Metabolism and Detoxification)

Aventurine: Page 60 (→ Immune System)

Zoisite: Page 56 (→ Metabolism, Immune System)

Zoisite with ruby: Page 57 (→ Immune System, Metabolism, Power and Vitality)

Ocean Jasper: Page 55 (→ Immune System, Detoxification, Regeneration)

Star Agate: Page 44 (→ Immune System, Protection and Boundary Setting)

Opalized Petrified Wood: Page 54 (→ Metabolism and Detoxification)

Jade (Jadeite/Nephrite): Page 58 (→ Metabolism)

Green Tourmaline (Verdelite): Page 60 (→ Metabolism, Autonomic Nervous System)

Choosing the Right Crystal

An Analytical Approach

What sort of problems are you experiencing? If several, which are the most prominent? Begin by narrowing down the list of possible crystals to use by choosing one of the general section headings (*Regeneration, Harmonization and Balance...*). Turn to the relevant section and look for the crystal that best fits your symptoms. You will find an index of issues or symptoms and their suitable crystals on pages 76–77.

An Intuitive Approach

As we stated at the beginning of the book, the healing power of crystals lies in their energetic effects. The phenomenon of resonance plays a major role in this.

Resonance is derived from the Latin *resonare*, which means to vibrate with or to sound in response. For example, if there are two guitars in the same room and you pluck a string on the first guitar, the same string on the second guitar will begin to resonate and even produce a sound, providing both strings are tuned to the same note. One string is stimulating the other to vibrate along with it and so is in a state of resonance.

The same applies to living organisms and energetic healing. For example, if the vibration of a healing substance corresponds exactly with an illness or a symptom, then a good effect can be achieved, even with vibrations that are so subtle they are not physically measurable. Homeopathy and Bach Flower Remedies are based on this principle. The greatest effect and the deepest healing are achieved when the vibrations of the healing substance correspond with the mood, character, and spiritual and mental condition of the patient at the time.

This is when the strongest possible resonance can be achieved—on physical, mental, and spiritual levels.

You can make use of the resonance principle to find the right crystal (or crystals) for your own issues. Everyone can sense resonance. It is the feeling of being addressed by or attracted to something intuitively and spontaneously, without thinking about it. You might suddenly have a strong feeling and think to yourself "Yes, that's it!" or just find something attractive or interesting. Perhaps you stop instinctively at the sight of something or at a particular sentence in a book, and only then begin to think about it. Or you might feel the resonance physically, as a sensation in your very core or your heart.

Simply follow this feeling or spontaneous moment of interest. Perhaps you have experienced such a moment while reading this book. Try and remember which crystals or keywords caught your interest.

If you can't remember anything specifically, look through all the general section headings again and choose one or two of them. Then read a few of the crystals' descriptions and be alert to which crystal appeals spontaneously to you.

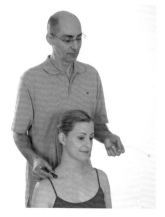
Testing with a single dowsing rod

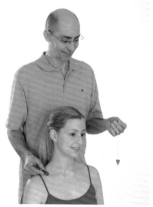
Testing with a pendulum

A pendulum or a single dowsing rod can help to make the resonance visible. This is especially meaningful if you have not yet experienced being guided by your intuition and the subtle signals that your body and soul send out. Working with a pendulum or a dowsing rod is a great way of accessing your intuition when trying to choose the right crystal.

The best results are achieved with a combination of the analytical and intuitive approaches. If both results converge, you will have found the ideal crystal to use.

Sometimes this will be quite easy and you will immediately know which crystal is needed, but other times it may be difficult to set priorities and many different crystals will appear to fit the situation. Then it may make sense to enlist the help of a professional crystal consultant.

Applying Crystals

There are many ways to use the power of crystals. For the purposes outlined in this book, we recommend wearing the relevant crystal for a time in direct contact with the skin. For example, a tumbled or raw crystal can be applied to the skin or you can wear it as a pendant or in a necklace. The length of time that it should be applied varies in individual cases and also depends on the type of crystal being used. The effects of some crystals may be felt relatively quickly, while others have to be worn for a longer period in order to take effect.

Generally speaking, the crystal should be worn long enough for the symptoms to disappear, or for as long as you feel comfortable wearing it. Sometimes a crystal just seems to vanish or is lost, or you forget about it, which probably indicates that it has now done its job.

Cleansing

Crystals that are worn for long periods of time should be cleansed on a regular basis, both physically and energetically. To cleanse a crystal physically, place it under running water for a while. For energetic cleansing, place it upon or within a piece of amethyst or smoky crystal druse. This has the additional advantage of also recharging it energetically.

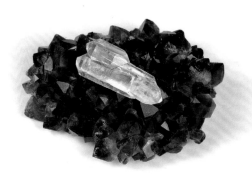

Alternatively, you can cleanse crystals with salt. Place the crystal in a shallow dish with dry salt crystals for 3–4 hours (no longer!). Most crystals cope well with this, but occasionally the procedure may lead to a dulling of the surface of crystals that are polished and shiny. If you want to be absolutely certain no harm will come to your crystals, place them in a small dish and then place that dish in a larger one containing the salt. In this way the crystals have no direct contact with the salt, but are cleansed nevertheless. More detailed information on cleansing and recharging crystals can be found in the small guide *Purifying Crystals* by Michael Gienger, which is available from Earthdancer Books.

Crystal-Based Anti-interference Devices

Many helpful devices are available that use crystals to eliminate interference caused by geopathic radiation or electromagnetic radiation. They usually contain tumbled crystals or granulates made of the classic anti-interference crystals, or combinations of these. They include mats filled with granulated tourmaline for placing under the bed, pyramids holding crystals, raw crystals, pendants and amulets, among others.

Some of these items have been produced with good intentions, but unfortunately many are inferior or fakes, using the cheapest tumbled crystal mixture, glued together, perhaps also designed to be plugged into the electricity supply and sold for a high price.

Many such items are elaborate and expensive, and in my opinion do not represent value for money. It makes much more sense to invest in a building biology investigation instead of spending money on expensive and often ineffective anti-interference devices.

As a rule, a raw or tumbled crystal will achieve the desired effect on an energetic level. If something more is required, a necklace will often work very well. Using more crystals or spending more money does not necessarily translate into greater effectiveness. As crystals are not actually able to reduce the amount of radiation being emitted or shield you from it, but instead work on an energetic level, elaborate crystal combinations or placing large numbers of crystals under the bed will not provide any more protection than one very ordinary, good-quality crystal.

Index of Conditions and Crystals

Acidosis (excess of acid in the body): charoite, emerald, heliotrope, mica, serpentine, turquoise, zoisite

Adrenal glands: jade, ruby

Allergies: aventurine, chrysoprase

Autonomic nervous system: amazonite, amber, ametrine, charoite, sunstone, tourmaline

Blood: garnet, jasper (brown and yellow), opalite

Boundary setting: agate, aventurine, black tourmaline, heliotrope, jade, mica, serpentine, turquoise

Circulation: garnet, red chalcedony, red jasper, ruby, tiger iron

Clogged tissues: chalcedony, chrysoprase, opalite, opalized petrified wood

Cramp: amazonite, charoite, serpentine, turquoise

Detoxification: aventurine, copper chalcedony, dendritic agate, dendritic chalcedony, chrysoprase, emerald, green garnet, green tourmaline, heliotrope, jade, mica, ocean jasper, opalite, opalized petrified wood, star agate, turquoise, zoisite

Digestion: epidote, jasper (brown and yellow)

Drive: ametrine, charoite, garnet, jade, jasper, mookaite, red jasper, ruby

Energy: clear quartz, tiger iron, turquoise

Exhaustion: epidote, heliotrope, ruby, tiger iron, turquoise

Harmonization and balance: amazonite, ametrine, aventurine, emerald, jade, mookaite, rose quartz, serpentine, sunstone, tourmaline

Heart: aventurine, charoite, green tourmaline, pink chalcedony, rose quartz

Identity: mica, turquoise

Immune system: chalcedony, dendritic agate, emerald, epidote, fuchsite, fuchsite with ruby, garnet, heliotrope, jasper, mookaite, ocean jasper, ruby, star agate, tourmaline, zoisite

Inflammation: emerald, green garnet, heliotrope, turquoise, zoisite

Kidneys: amber, jade, serpentine

Liver: amber, chrysoprase, emerald, epidote, garnet, red tourmaline, star agate

Lungs: blue chalcedony, opalite

Lymph: chalcedony, chrysoprase, heliotrope

Metabolism: amazonite, ametrine, chrysoprase, dendritic agate, garnet, heliotrope, opalite, petrified wood, ruby, serpentine, tourmaline, turquoise

Mood swings: amazonite, serpentine, turquoise

Mucus membranes: amber, opalite

Nasal sinus cavities: emerald

Nerves: amazonite, jade, lepidolite, petrified wood, smoky quartz, tourmaline

Nervousness: aventurine, heliotrope, serpentine

Pain: clear quartz, lepidolite, smoky quartz, tourmaline, tourmaline quartz, turquoise

Power and vitality: epidote, fuchsite with ruby, garnet, hematite, mookaite, red jasper, ruby, tiger iron

Protection: agate, aventurine, black tourmaline, heliotrope, jade, mica, serpentine, turquoise

Reality, sense of: agate, epidote, petrified wood

Regeneration: brown tourmaline, emerald, epidote, garnet, ocean jasper, zoisite, zoisite with ruby

Relaxation: amazonite, aventurine, smoky quartz

Self-confidence: amber, ruby, sunstone

Self-determination: amazonite, ametrine, turquoise, zoisite

Sleep: aventurine, ocean jasper, tektite

Spleen: amber, mookaite, red tourmaline, ruby

Stability: agate, amber, dendritic agate, mookaite, ocean jasper, petrified wood, star agate

Stamina: dendritic agate, garnet, jasper (red, brown, and yellow), mookaite, tiger iron

Stress: aventurine, black tourmaline, charoite, smoky quartz, serpentine

Tiredness: hematite, heliotrope, ruby, tiger iron

Trust: amazonite, amber, chrysoprase, dendritic agate, garnet, lepidolite, pink chalcedony

Willpower: garnet, mookaite, red jasper, ruby

Wound healing: amber, garnet

Crystals Index

Thanks

Thank you to Dagmar Fleck and Michael Gienger for their valuable support in the selection and classification of suitable crystals. This small book could not have been written without their generosity and willingness to share their expansive knowledge and long experience of crystal healing.

Useful Addresses for Building Biology

Building biology (or Baubiologie as it originated in Germany) is a field of building science that investigates the indoor living environment for a variety of irritants. Practitioners consider the built environment as something with which the occupants interact, and believe its functioning can produce a restful or stressful environment. The major areas focused on by building biologists are building materials/process, indoor air quality (IAQ), and electromagnetic fields (EMFs).

Institute for Bau-Biologie & Ecology
P.O. Box 738
Lyles, TN 37098
United States
Tel: 1-866-960-0333 (toll-free in US & Canada)
https://buildingbiologyinstitute.org

Building Biology Environmental Consultant (IBN)
Rainbow Consulting, Katharina Gustavs
5237 Mt. Matheson Rd., Sooke BC V9Z 1C4, Canada
Tel: 250-642-2774
info@buildingbiology.ca
www.buildingbiology.ca

The Building Biology Association UK
18 Market Place
Bideford
Devon EX39 2DR
Tel: 01237 474952
bba@buildingbiology.co.uk
www.buildingbiology.co.uk

Picture credits

Photos.com/Dragon Design: 8.

Shutterstock.com: 12–13; 17: metamorworks; 20: nmedia; 24: Roman Samsonov; 27: tomertu; 33: Nastya22.

Shutterstock/Dragon Design: 22, 31.

Barbara Newerla: 9, 36, 38, 40, 43, 45 top, 48, 49, 50, 51 top, 51 btm., 52, 53 btm., 56 top, 60, 63, 67, 68 top.

Karola Sieber: 34, 41, 47, 51 mid., 53 top, 54, 55, 56 btm., 58, 62 btm., 65 btm., 66, 68 btm.

Dragon Design: 35.

Ines Blersch: 44, 45 btm., 46, 57, 59, 62 top, 65 top, 71, 73.

For further information and to request a book catalog contact:
Inner Traditions, One Park Street, Rochester, Vermont 05767

Earthdancer Books is an Inner Traditions imprint.
Phone: +1-800-246-8648, customerservice@innertraditions.com
www.earthdancerbooks.com • www.innertraditions.com

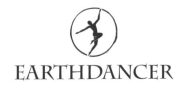

EARTHDANCER

AN INNER TRADITIONS IMPRINT